Mediterranean Diet Cookbook for Beginners 2021

Boost your Health with 50 Recipes Easy and Quick to Prepare

By Dianne Wade

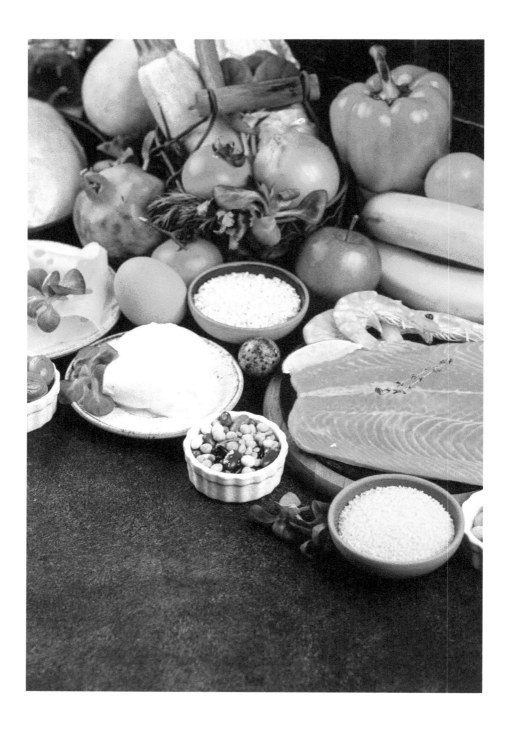

Table of Contents

Chapter 7: Dessert Recipes *98*

Introduction

Mediterranean diet is based on the eating habits of the inhabitants of the regions along the Mediterranean Sea, mostly from Italy, Spain and Greece; it is considered more a life style then a diet, in fact it also promotes physical activity and proper liquid (mostly water) consumption.

Depending on fresh seasonal local foods there are no strict rules, because of the many cultural differences, but there are some common factors.

Mediterranean diet has become famous for its ability to reduce heart disease and obesity, thanks to the low consumption of unhealthy fats that increase blood glucose.

Mediterranean diet is mostly plant based, so it's rich of antioxidants; vegetables, fruits like apple and grapes, olive oil, whole grains, herbs, beans and nuts are consumed in large quantities.

Moderate amounts of poultry, eggs, dairy and seafood are also common aliments, accompanied by a little bit of red wine (some studies say that in small amount it helps to stay healthy).

Red meat and sweets like cookies and cakes are accepted but are more limited in quantity.

Foods to avoid:

- refined grains, such as white bread and pasta
- dough containing white flour refined oils (even canola oil and soybean oil)
- foods with added sugars (like pastries, sodas, and candies)
- processed meats processed or packaged foods

Chapter 1: Breakfast and Snack Recipes

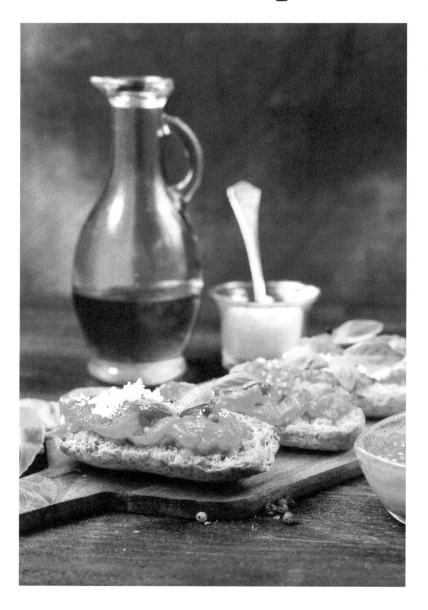

Sun-dried Tomatoes Oatmeal

Preparation: 10 min | Cooking: 25 min | Servings: 4

Ingredients

- 3 cups water
- 1 cup almond milk
- 1 tablespoon olive oil
- 1 cup steel-cut oats
- ¼ cup sun-dried tomatoes, chopped

Directions

1. In a pan, scourge water with the milk, bring to a boil over medium heat.
2. Meanwhile, pre-heat pan with the oil over medium-high heat, add the oats, cook them for about 2 min and transfer m to the pan with the milk.
3. Stir the oats, add the tomatoes and simmer over medium heat for 23 min.
4. Divide the mix into bowls, sprinkle the red pepper flakes on top and serve for breakfast.

Nutrition: 170 calories; 17.8g fat; 1.5g protein

Quinoa Muffins

Preparation: 10 min | Cooking: 30 min | Servings: 12

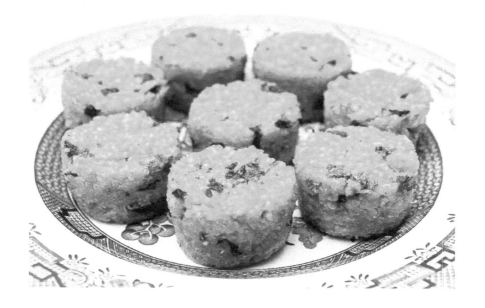

Ingredients

- 6 eggs, whisked
- 1 cup Swiss cheese, grated
- 1 small yellow onion, chopped
- 1 cup quinoa, white mushrooms
- ½ cup sun-dried tomatoes, chopped

Directions

1. In a bowl, combine the eggs with salt, pepper and the rest of the ingredients and whisk well.
2. Divide this into a silicone muffin pan, bake at 350 degrees F for 30 min and serve for breakfast.

Nutrition: 123 calories; 5.6g fat; 7.5g protein

Watermelon "Pizza"

Preparation: 10 min | Cooking: 0 min | Servings: 4

Ingredients

- 1 watermelon slice cut 1-inch thick and then from the center cut into 4 wedges resembling pizza slices
- 6 kalamata olives, pitted and sliced
- 1-ounce feta cheese, crumbled
- ½ tablespoon balsamic vinegar
- 1 teaspoon mint, chopped

Directions

1. Arrange the watermelon "pizza" on a plate, sprinkle the olives and the rest of the ingredients on each slice and serve right away for breakfast.

Nutrition: 90 calories; 3g fat; 2g protein

Cheesy Yogurt

Preparation: 4 hs and 5 min | Cooking: 0 min | Servings: 4

Ingredients

- 1 cup Greek yogurt
- 1 tablespoon honey
- ½ cup feta cheese, crumbled

Directions

1. In a blender, combine the yogurt with the honey and the cheese and pulse well.
2. Divide into bowls and freeze for 4 hs before serving for breakfast.

Nutrition: 161 calories; 10g fat; 6.6g protein

Cauliflower Fritters

Preparation: 10 min | Cooking: 50 min | Servings: 4

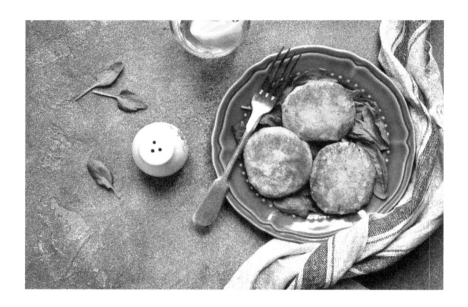

Ingredients

- 30 ounces canned chickpeas, drained and rinsed
- 2 and ½ tablespoons olive oil
- 1 small yellow onion, chopped
- 2 cups cauliflower florets chopped
- 2 tablespoons garlic, minced

Directions

1. Lay out half of the chickpeas on a baking sheet lined with parchment pepper, pour in 1 tablespoon oil, season well, toss and bake at 400 degrees F for 30 min.
2. Transfer the chickpeas to a food processor, pulse well and put the mix into a bowl.
3. Heat up a pan with the ½ tablespoon oil over medium-high heat, add the garlic and the onion and sauté for 3 min.
4. Add the cauliflower, cook for 6 min more, transfer this to a blender, add the rest of the chickpeas, pulse, pour over the crispy chickpeas mix from the bowl, stir and shape medium fritters out of this mix.
5. Heat up a pan with the rest of the oil over medium-high heat, add the fritters, cook them for 6 min on both side and serve for breakfast.

Nutrition: 333 calories; 12.6g fat; 13.6g protein

Corn and Shrimp Salad

Preparation: 10 min | Cooking: 10 min | Servings: 4

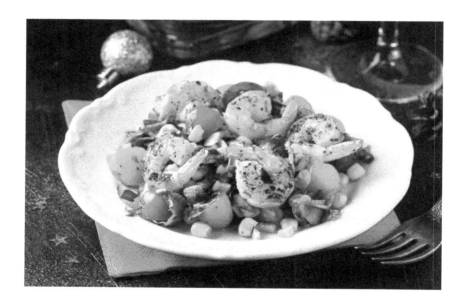

Ingredients

- 4 ears of sweet corn, husked
- 1 avocado, peeled, pitted and chopped
- ½ cup basil, chopped
- 1-pound shrimp, peeled and deveined
- 1 and ½ cups cherry tomatoes, halved

Directions

1. Put the corn in a pot, boil water and cover, over medium heat for 6 min, drain, cool down, cut corn from the cob and put it in a bowl.
2. Thread the shrimp onto skewers and brush with some of the oil.
3. Situate the skewers on the prepared grill, cook over medium heat for 2 min on each side, remove from skewers and add over the corn.
4. Place the rest of the ingredients to the bowl, toss, divide between plates and serve for breakfast.

Nutrition: 371 calories; 22g fat; 23g protein

Cottage Cheese and Berries Omelet

Preparation: 5 min | Cooking: 4 min | Servings: 1

Ingredients

- 1 egg, whisked
- 1 teaspoon cinnamon powder
- 1 tablespoon almond milk
- 3 ounces cottage cheese
- 4 ounces blueberries

Directions

1. Scourge egg with the rest of the ingredients except the oil and toss.
2. Preheat pan with the oil over medium heat, add the eggs mix, spread, cook for 4 min on both sides, then serve.

Nutrition: 190 calories; 8g fat; 2g protein

Salmon Frittata

Preparation: 5 min | Cooking: 27 min | Servings: 4

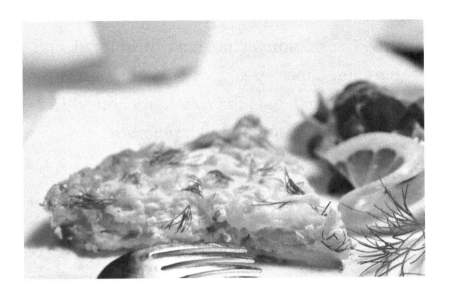

Ingredients

- 1-pound gold potatoes, roughly cubed
- 1 tablespoon olive oil
- 2 salmon fillets, skinless and boneless
- 8 eggs, whisked
- 1 teaspoon mint, chopped

Directions

1. Put the potatoes in a boiling water at medium heat, then cook for 12 min, drain and transfer to a bowl.
2. Spread the salmon on a baking sheet lined with parchment paper, grease with cooking spray, broil at medium-high heat for 10 min on both sides, cool down, flake and put in a separate bowl.
3. Warm up a pan with the oil over medium heat, add the potatoes, salmon, and the rest of the ingredients excluding the eggs and toss.
4. Add the eggs on top, put the lid on and cook over medium heat for 10 min.
5. Divide the salmon between plates and serve.

Nutrition: 289 calories; 11g fat; 4g protein

Avocado and Olive Paste on Toasted Rye Bread

Preparation: 5 min | Cooking: 0 minute| Servings: 4

Ingredients

- 1 avocado, halved, peeled and finely chopped
- 1 tbsp green onions, finely chopped
- 2 tbsp green olive paste
- 4 lettuce leaves
- 1 tbsp lemon juice

Directions

1. Crush avocados with a fork or potato masher until almost smooth. Add the onions, green olive paste and lemon juice. Season with salt and pepper to taste. Stir to combine.
2. Toast 4 slices of rye bread until golden. Spoon 1/4 of the avocado mixture onto each slice of bread, top with a lettuce leaf and serve.

Nutrition: 291 calories; 13g fat; 3g protein

Chapter 2: Lunch & Dinner Recipes

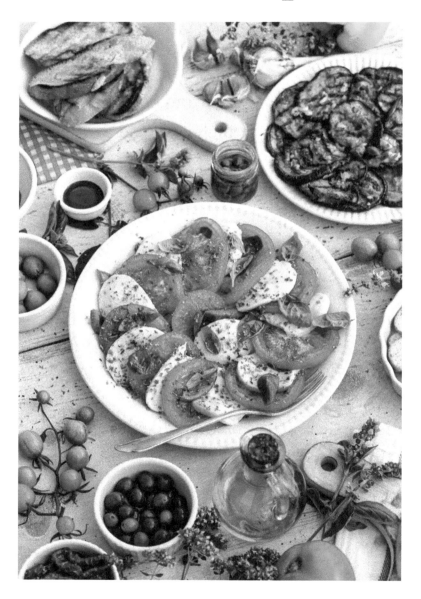

Vegetable Turkey Casserole

Servings: 8 | Cooking: 1 ¼ Hours

Ingredients

- 3 tablespoons olive oil
- 2 pounds turkey breasts, cubed
- 1 sweet onion, chopped
- 3 carrots, sliced
- 2 celery stalks, sliced
- 2 garlic cloves, chopped
- ½ teaspoon cumin powder
- ½ teaspoon dried thyme
- 2 cans diced tomatoes
- 1 cup chicken stock
- 1 bay leaf
- Salt and pepper to taste

Directions

1. Heat the oil in a deep heavy pot and stir in the turkey.

2. Cook for 5 minutes until golden on all sides then add the onion, carrot, celery and garlic. Cook for 5 more minutes then add the rest of the ingredients.
3. Season with salt and pepper and cook in the preheated oven at 350F for 40 minutes.
4. Serve the casserole warm and fresh.

Nutrition: Calories:186 Fat:7.3g Protein:20.1g Carbohydrates:9.9g

Mediterranean Grilled Pork With Tomato Salsa

Servings: 4 | Cooking: 1 Hour

Ingredients

- 4 pork chops
- 1 teaspoon dried oregano
- 1 teaspoon dried basil
- 1 teaspoon dried marjoram
- Salt and pepper to taste
- 4 tomatoes, peeled and diced
- 1 jalapeno, chopped
- 1 shallot, chopped
- 2 garlic cloves, minced
- 1 green onion, chopped
- 2 tablespoons chopped parsley
- 1 tablespoon lemon juice

Directions

1. Season with salt and pepper, oregano, basil and marjoram.

27

2. Heat a grill pan over medium flame and place the pork chops on the grill.
3. Cook on each side for 5-6 minutes.
4. For the salsa, mix the tomatoes, jalapeno, shallot, garlic, onion and parsley. Add salt and pepper to taste. Add the lemon juice as well.
5. Serve the pork chops with salsa.

Nutrition: Calories:286 Fat:20.3g Protein:19.4g Carbohydrates:6.3g

Beef And Macaroni Soup

Servings: 6 | Cooking: 30 min

Ingredients

- ½ cup elbow macaroni
- 1 teaspoon coconut oil
- 1/3 teaspoon minced garlic
- 2 oz yellow onion, diced
- 1 ½ cup ground beef
- ½ teaspoon dried oregano
- ½ teaspoon dried thyme
- 1 teaspoon salt
- 1 teaspoon chili flakes
- 3 oz Mozzarella, shredded
- 1 teaspoon dried basil
- 5 cups beef broth
- 1 tablespoon cream cheese
- 1 cup water, for cooking macaroni

Directions

1. Pour water in the pan and bring it to boil.

2. Add elbow macaroni and cook them according to the manufacturer directions.
3. Then drain water from the cooked elbow macaroni.
4. Put coconut oil in the big pot and melt it.
5. Add minced garlic, yellow onion, ground beef, dried oregano, dried thyme, salt, chili flakes, and dried basil.
6. Cook the ingredients for 10 minutes over the medium-low heat. Stir the mixture from time to time.
7. Add beef broth and cream cheese. Stir the soup until it is homogenous.
8. Cook the soup for 10 minutes.
9. Then add cooked elbow macaroni and stir well.
10. Bring the soup to boil and remove from the heat.
11. Ladle the cooked soup in the serving bowls and garnish with Mozzarella.

Nutrition: calories 180; fat 9.2; fiber 0.5; carbs 7.6; protein 15.7

Provencal Beef Stew

Servings: 8 | Cooking: 1 ½ Hours

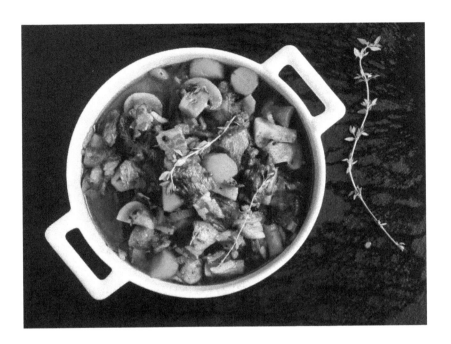

Ingredients

- 3 tablespoons olive oil
- 2 pounds beef roast, cubed
- 2 sweet onions, chopped
- 4 garlic cloves, chopped
- 2 carrots, diced
- 2 celery stalks, diced
- 1 can diced tomatoes

- 2 tomatoes, peeled and diced
- 1 cup vegetable stock
- 1 jalapeno, chopped
- 1 bay leaf
- 1 thyme sprig
- Salt and pepper to taste

Directions

1. Heat the oil in a skillet and stir in the beef. Cook for 10 minutes on all sides.
2. Add the onions and garlic and cook for 5 more minutes.
3. Stir in the remaining ingredients and season with salt and pepper.
4. Place a lid on and cook on low heat for 1 hour.
5. Serve the stew warm and fresh.

Nutrition: Calories:284 Fat:12.5g Protein:35.4g Carbohydrates:6.5g

Greek Beef Meatballs

Servings: 8 | Cooking: 1 Hour

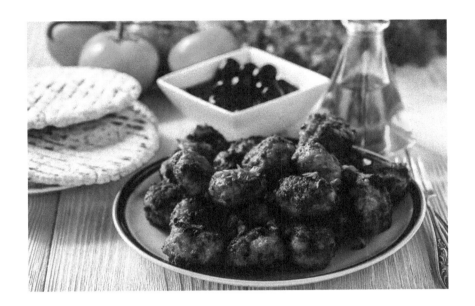

Ingredients

- 2 pounds ground beef
- 6 garlic cloves, minced
- 1 teaspoon dried mint
- 1 teaspoon dried oregano
- 1 shallot, finely chopped
- 1 carrot, grated
- 1 egg
- 1 tablespoon tomato paste

33

- 3 tablespoons chopped parsley
- Salt and pepper to taste

Directions

1. Combine all the ingredients in a bowl and mix well.
2. Season with salt and pepper then form small meatballs and place them in a baking tray lined with baking paper.
3. Bake in the preheated oven at 350F for 25 minutes.
4. Serve the meatballs warm and fresh.

Nutrition: Calories:229 Fat:7.7g Protein:35.5g Carbohydrates:2.4g

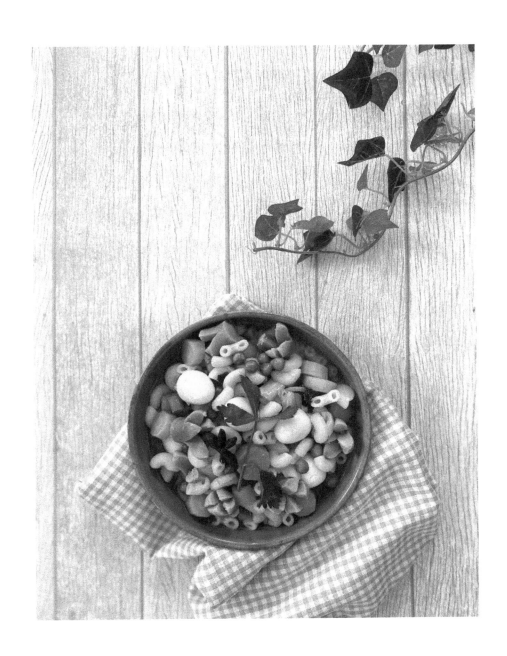

Chapter 3: Meat Recipes

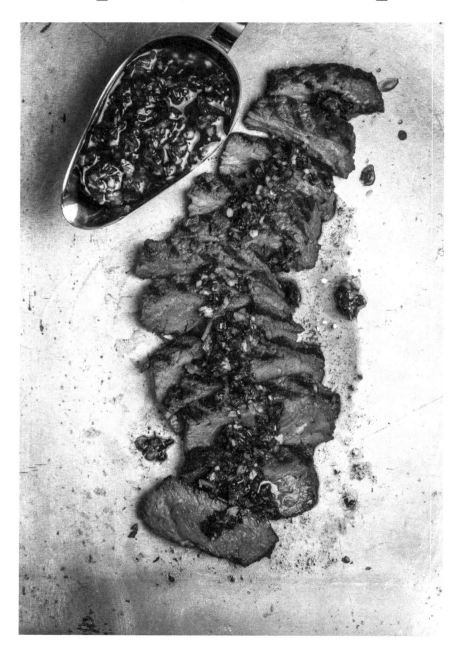

Pork Kebabs

Servings: 6 | Cooking: 14 min

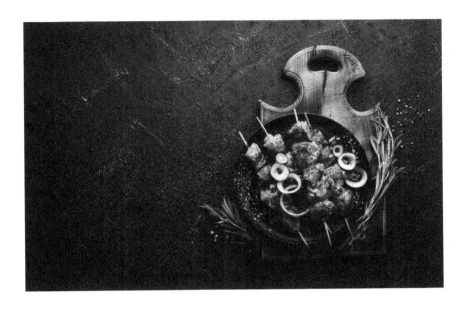

Ingredients

- 1 yellow onion, chopped
- 1 pound pork meat, ground
- 3 tablespoons cilantro, chopped
- 1 tablespoon lime juice
- 1 garlic clove, minced
- 2 teaspoon oregano, dried
- Salt and black pepper to the taste
- A drizzle of olive oil

37

Directions

1. In a bowl, mix the pork with the other ingredients except the oil, stir well and shape medium kebabs out of this mix.
2. Divide the kebabs on skewers, and brush them with a drizzle of oil.
3. Place the kebabs on your preheated grill and cook over medium heat for 7 minutes on each side.
4. Divide the kebabs between plates and serve with a side salad.

Nutrition: calories 229; fat 14; fiber 8.3; carbs 15.5; protein 12.4

Vegetable Lover's Chicken Soup

Servings: 4 | Cooking: 20 min

Ingredients

- 1 ½ cups baby spinach
- 2 tbsp orzo (tiny pasta)
- ¼ cup dry white wine
- 1 14oz low sodium chicken broth
- 2 plum tomatoes, chopped
- 1/8 tsp salt
- ½ tsp Italian seasoning
- 1 large shallot, chopped
- 1 small zucchini, diced
- 8-oz chicken tenders
- 1 tbsp extra virgin olive oil

Directions

1. In a large saucepan, heat oil over medium heat and add the chicken. Stir occasionally for 8 minutes until browned. Transfer in a plate. Set aside.
2. In the same saucepan, add the zucchini, Italian seasoning, shallot and salt and stir often until the vegetables are softened, around 4 minutes.

3. Add the tomatoes, wine, broth and orzo and increase the heat to high to bring the mixture to boil. Reduce the heat and simmer.
4. Add the cooked chicken and stir in the spinach last.
5. Serve hot.

Nutrition: Calories: 207; Carbs: 14.8g; Protein: 12.2g; Fat: 11.4g

Lemony Lamb And Potatoes

Servings: 4 | Cooking: 2 Hours And 10 min

Ingredients

- 2 pound lamb meat, cubed
- 2 tablespoons olive oil
- 2 springs rosemary, chopped
- 2 tablespoons parsley, chopped
- 1 tablespoon lemon rind, grated
- 3 garlic cloves, minced
- 2 tablespoons lemon juice
- 2 pounds baby potatoes, scrubbed and halved
- 1 cup veggie stock

Directions

1. In a roasting pan, combine the meat with the oil and the rest of the ingredients, introduce in the oven and bake at 400 degrees F for 2 hours and 10 minutes.
2. Divide the mix between plates and serve.

Nutrition: calories 302; fat 15.2; fiber 10.6; carbs 23.3; protein 15.2

Cumin Lamb Mix

Servings: 2 | Cooking: 10 min

Ingredients

- 2 lamb chops (3.5 oz each)
- 1 tablespoon olive oil
- 1 teaspoon ground cumin
- ½ teaspoon salt

Directions

1. Rub the lamb chops with ground cumin and salt.
2. Then sprinkle them with olive oil.
3. Let the meat marinate for 10 minutes.
4. After this, preheat the skillet well.
5. Place the lamb chops in the skillet and roast them for 10 minutes. Flip the meat on another side from time to time to avoid burning.

Nutrition: calories 384; fat 33.2; fiber 0.1; carbs 0.5; protein 19.2

Almond Lamb Chops

Servings: 4 | Cooking: 20 min

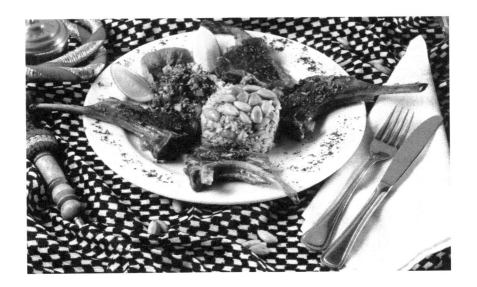

Ingredients

- 1 teaspoon almond butter
- 2 teaspoons minced garlic
- 1 teaspoon butter, softened
- ½ teaspoon salt
- ½ teaspoon chili flakes
- ½ teaspoon ground paprika
- 12 oz lamb chop

Directions

1. Churn together minced garlic, butter, salt, chili flakes, and ground paprika.
2. Carefully rub every lamb chop with the garlic mixture.
3. Toss almond butter in the skillet and melt it.
4. Place the lamb chops in the melted almond butter and roast them for 20 minutes (for 10 minutes from each side) over the medium-low heat.

Nutrition: calories 194; fat 9.5; fiber 0.5; carbs 1.4; protein 24.9

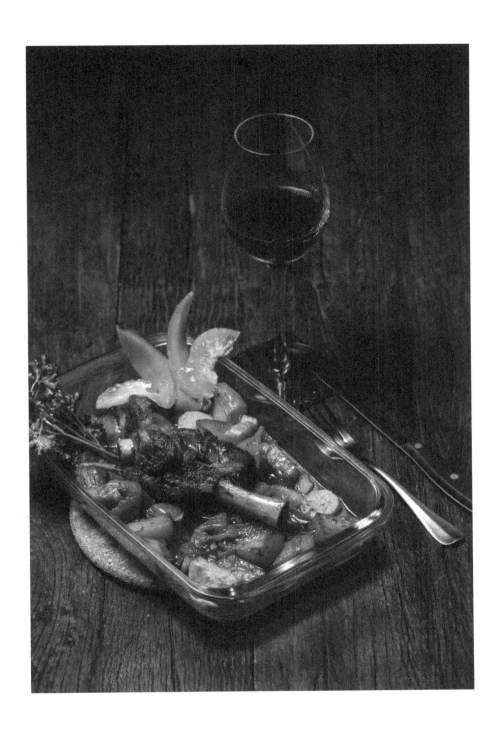

Chapter 4: Poultry Recipes

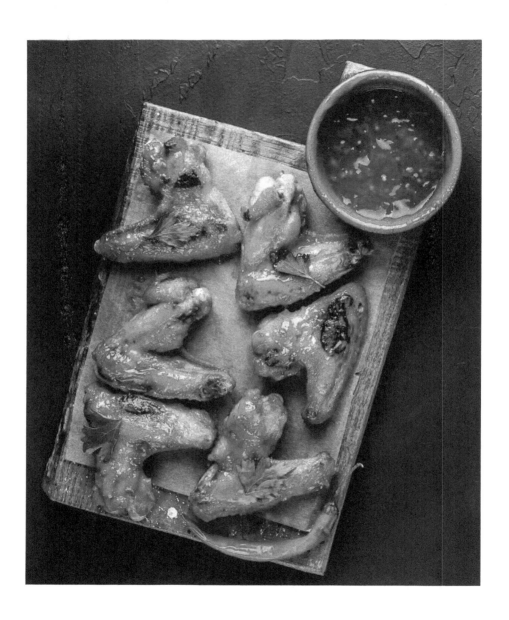

Lemon Chicken Mix

Servings: 2 | Cooking: 10 min

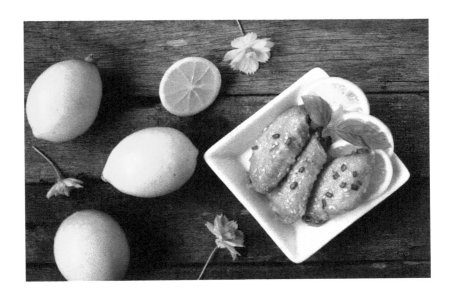

Ingredients

- 8 oz chicken breast, skinless, boneless
- 1 teaspoon Cajun seasoning
- 1 teaspoon balsamic vinegar
- 1 teaspoon olive oil
- 1 teaspoon lemon juice

Directions

1. Cut the chicken breast on the halves and sprinkle with Cajun seasoning.
2. Then sprinkle the poultry with olive oil and lemon juice.
3. Then sprinkle the chicken breast with the balsamic vinegar.
4. Preheat the grill to 385F.
5. Grill the chicken breast halves for 5 minutes from each side.
6. Slice Cajun chicken and place in the serving plate.

Nutrition: calories 150; fat 5.2; fiber 0; carbs 0.1; protein 24.1

Turkey And Chickpeas

Servings: 4 | Cooking: 5 Hours

Ingredients

- 2 tablespoons avocado oil
- 1 big turkey breast, skinless, boneless and roughly cubed
- Salt and black pepper to the taste
- 1 red onion, chopped
- 15 ounces canned chickpeas, drained and rinsed
- 15 ounces canned tomatoes, chopped
- 1 cup kalamata olives, pitted and halved
- 2 tablespoons lime juice
- 1 teaspoon oregano, dried

Directions

1. Heat up a pan with the oil over medium-high heat, add the meat and the onion, brown for 5 minutes and transfer to a slow cooker.
2. Add the rest of the ingredients, put the lid on and cook on High for 5 hours.
3. Divide between plates and serve right away!

Nutrition: calories 352; fat 14.4; fiber 11.8; carbs 25.1; protein 26.4

Cardamom Chicken And Apricot Sauce

Servings: 4 | Cooking: 7 Hours

Ingredients

- Juice of ½ lemon
- Zest of ½ lemon, grated
- 2 teaspoons cardamom, ground
- Salt and black pepper to the taste
- 2 chicken breasts, skinless, boneless and halved
- 2 tablespoons olive oil
- 2 spring onions, chopped
- 2 tablespoons tomato paste
- 2 garlic cloves, minced
- 1 cup apricot juice
- ½ cup chicken stock
- ¼ cup cilantro, chopped

Directions

1. In your slow cooker, combine the chicken with the lemon juice, lemon zest and the other ingredients except the cilantro, toss, put the lid on and cook on Low for 7 hours.

2. Divide the mix between plates, sprinkle the cilantro on top and serve.

Nutrition: calories 323; fat 12; fiber 11; carbs 23.8; protein 16.4

Chicken and Artichokes

Servings: 4 | Cooking: 20 min

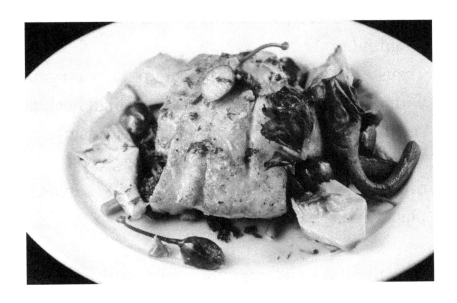

Ingredients

- 2 pounds chicken breast, skinless, boneless and sliced
- A pinch of salt and black pepper
- 4 tablespoons olive oil
- 8 ounces canned roasted artichoke hearts, drained
- 6 ounces sun-dried tomatoes, chopped
- 3 tablespoons capers, drained
- 2 tablespoons lemon juice

Directions

1. Heat up a pan with half of the oil over medium-high heat, add the artichokes and the other ingredients except the chicken, stir and sauté for 10 minutes.
2. Transfer the mix to a bowl, heat up the pan again with the rest of the oil over medium-high heat, add the meat and cook for 4 minutes on each side.
3. Return the veggie mix to the pan, toss, cook everything for 2-3 minutes more, divide between plates and serve.

Nutrition: calories 552; fat 28; fiber 6; carbs 33; protein 43

Buttery Chicken Spread

Servings: 6 | Cooking: 20 min

Ingredients

- 8 oz chicken liver
- 3 tablespoon butter
- 1 white onion, chopped
- 1 bay leaf
- 1 teaspoon salt
- ½ teaspoon ground black pepper
- ½ cup of water

Directions

1. Place the chicken liver in the saucepan.
2. Add onion, bay leaf, salt, ground black pepper, and water.
3. Mix up the mixture and close the lid.
4. Cook the liver mixture for 20 minutes over the medium heat.
5. Then transfer it in the blender and blend until smooth.
6. Add butter and mix up until it is melted.

7. Pour the pate mixture in the pate ramekin and refrigerate for 2 hours.

Nutrition: calories 122; fat 8.3; fiber 0.5; carbs 2.3; protein 9.5

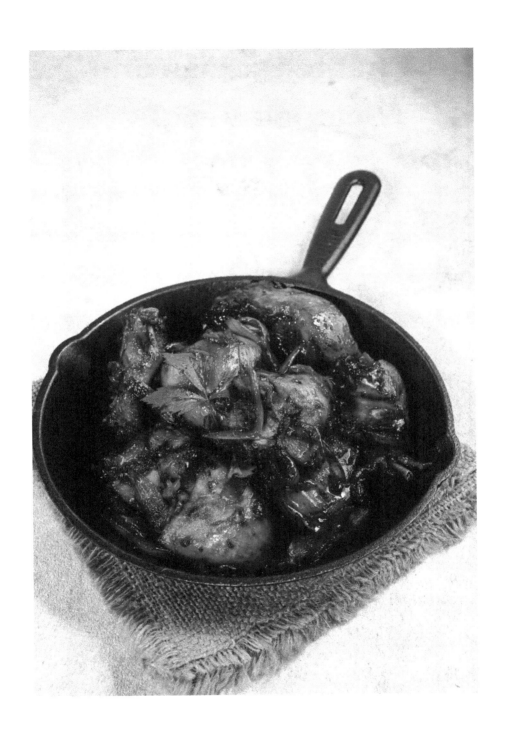

Chapter 5: Fish and Seafood Recipes

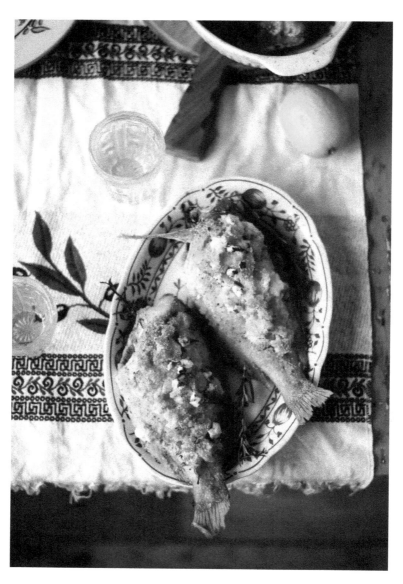

Cod And Mushrooms Mix

Servings: 4 | Cooking: 25 min

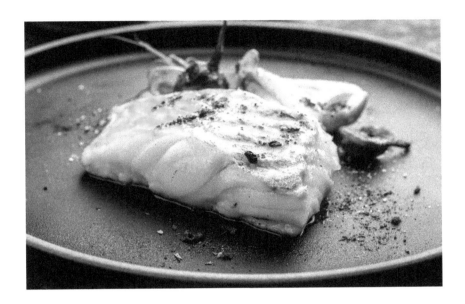

Ingredients

- 2 cod fillets, boneless
- 4 tablespoons olive oil
- 4 ounces mushrooms, sliced
- Sea salt and black pepper to the taste
- 12 cherry tomatoes, halved
- 8 ounces lettuce leaves, torn
- 1 avocado, pitted, peeled and cubed
- 1 red chili pepper, chopped

59

- 1 tablespoon cilantro, chopped
- 2 tablespoons balsamic vinegar
- 1 ounce feta cheese, crumbled

Directions

1. Put the fish in a roasting pan, brush it with 2 tablespoons oil, sprinkle salt and pepper all over and broil under medium-high heat for 15 minutes. Meanwhile, heat up a pan with the rest of the oil over medium heat, add the mushrooms, stir and sauté for 5 minutes.
2. Add the rest of the ingredients, toss, cook for 5 minutes more and divide between plates.
3. Top with the fish and serve right away.

Nutrition: calories 257; fat 10; fiber 3.1; carbs 24.3; protein 19.4

Baked Shrimp Mix

Servings: 4 | Cooking: 32 min

Ingredients

- 4 gold potatoes, peeled and sliced
- 2 fennel bulbs, trimmed and cut into wedges
- 2 shallots, chopped
- 2 garlic cloves, minced
- 3 tablespoons olive oil
- ½ cup kalamata olives, pitted and halved
- 2 pounds shrimp, peeled and deveined
- 1 teaspoon lemon zest, grated
- 2 teaspoons oregano, dried
- 4 ounces feta cheese, crumbled
- 2 tablespoons parsley, chopped

Directions

1. In a roasting pan, combine the potatoes with 2 tablespoons oil, garlic and the rest of the ingredients except the shrimp, toss, introduce in the oven and bake at 450 degrees F for 25 minutes.

2. Add the shrimp, toss, bake for 7 minutes more, divide between plates and serve.

Nutrition: calories 341; fat 19; fiber 9; carbs 34; protein 10

Lemon And Dates Barramundi

Servings: 2 | Cooking: 12 min

Ingredients

- 2 barramundi fillets, boneless
- 1 shallot, sliced
- 4 lemon slices
- Juice of ½ lemon
- Zest of 1 lemon, grated
- 2 tablespoons olive oil
- 6 ounces baby spinach
- ¼ cup almonds, chopped
- 4 dates, pitted and chopped
- ¼ cup parsley, chopped
- Salt and black pepper to the taste

Directions

1. Season the fish with salt and pepper and arrange on 2 parchment paper pieces.
2. Top the fish with the lemon slices, drizzle the lemon juice, and then top with the other ingredients except the oil.

3. Drizzle 1 tablespoon oil over each fish mix, wrap the parchment paper around the fish shaping to packets and arrange them on a baking sheet.
4. Bake at 400 degrees F for 12 minutes, cool the mix a bit, unfold, divide everything between plates and serve.

Nutrition: calories 232; fat 16.5; fiber 11.1; carbs 24.8; protein 6.5

Cheesy Crab And Lime Spread

Servings: 8 | Cooking: 25 min

Ingredients

- 1 pound crab meat, flaked
- 4 ounces cream cheese, soft
- 1 tablespoon chives, chopped
- 1 teaspoon lime juice
- 1 teaspoon lime zest, grated

Directions

1. In a baking dish greased with cooking spray, combine the crab with the rest of the ingredients and toss.
2. Introduce in the oven at 350 degrees F, bake for 25 minutes, divide into bowls and serve.

Nutrition: calories 284; fat 14.6; fiber 5.8; carbs 16.5; protein 15.4

Honey Lobster

Servings: 2 | Cooking: 10 min

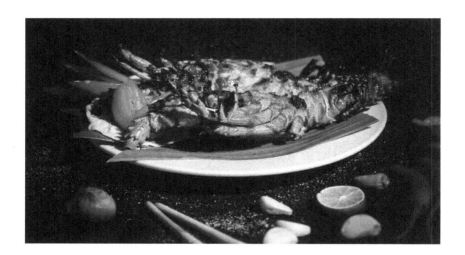

Ingredients

- 2 lobster tails
- 2 teaspoons butter, melted
- 1 teaspoon honey
- ¼ teaspoon ground paprika
- 1 teaspoon lemon juice
- ¼ teaspoon dried dill

Directions

1. Cut the top of the lobster tail shell to the tip of the tail with the help of the scissors. It will look like "lobster meat in a blanket".
2. Mix up together melted butter, honey, ground paprika, lemon juice, and dried dill.
3. Brush the lobster tails with butter mixture carefully from the top and down.
4. Preheat the oven to 365F.
5. Line the baking tray with parchment and arrange the lobster tails in it.
6. Bake the lobster tails for 10 minutes.

Nutrition: calories 91; fat 3.9; fiber 0.1 carbs 3.1; protein 0.1

Chapter 6: Salads & Side Dishes

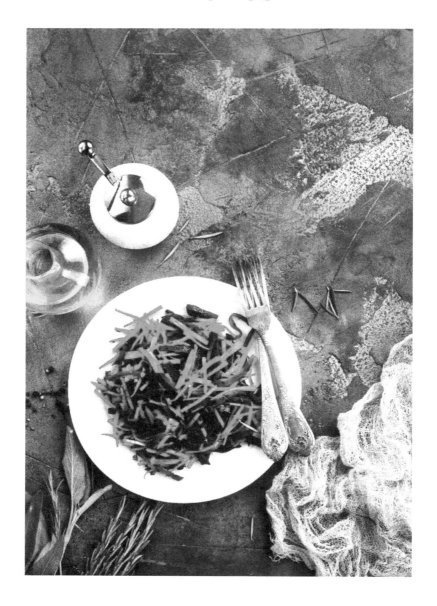

Vegetable-Stuffed Grape Leaves

Preparation: 50 min | Cooking: 45 min | Servings: 7

Ingredients

- 2 cups white rice, rinsed
- 2 large tomatoes, finely diced
- 1 (16-ounce) jar grape leaves
- 1 cup lemon juice
- 4 to 6 cups water

Directions

1. Incorporate rice, tomatoes, 1 onion, 1 green onion, 1 cup of parsley, 3 garlic cloves, salt, and black pepper.
2. Drain and rinse the grape leaves.
3. Prepare a large pot by placing a layer of grape leaves on the bottom. Lay each leaf flat and trim off any stems.
4. Place 2 tablespoons of the rice mixture at the base of each leaf. Fold over the sides, then roll as tight as possible. Situate the rolled grape leaves in the pot, lining up each rolled grape leaf. Continue to layer in the rolled grape leaves.

5. Gently pour the lemon juice and olive oil over the grape leaves, and add enough water to just cover the grape leaves by 1 inch.
6. Lay a heavy plate that is smaller than the opening of the pot upside down over the grape leaves. Cover the pot and cook the leaves over medium-low heat for 45 min. Let stand for 20 min before serving.
7. Serve warm or cold.

Nutrition: 532 Calories: 12g Protein: 80g Carbohydrates

Grilled Eggplant Rolls

Preparation: 30 min | Cooking: 10 min | Servings: 5

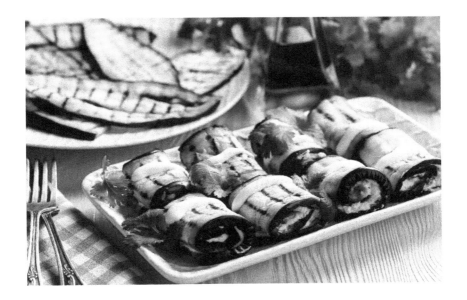

Ingredients

- 2 large eggplants
- 4 ounces goat cheese
- 1 cup ricotta
- ¼ cup fresh basil, finely chopped

Directions

1. Slice the tops of the eggplants off and cut the eggplants lengthwise into ¼-inch-thick slices.

Sprinkle the slices with the salt and place the eggplant in a colander for 15 to 20 min.

2. In a large bowl, combine the goat cheese, ricotta, basil, and pepper.
3. Preheat a grill, grill pan, or lightly oiled skillet on medium heat. Pat the eggplant slices dry using paper towel and lightly spray with olive oil spray. Place the eggplant on the grill, grill pan or skillet and cook for 3 min on each side.
4. Take out the eggplant from the heat and let cool for 5 min.
5. To roll, lay one eggplant slice flat, place a tablespoon of the cheese mixture at the base of the slice, and roll up. Serve immediately or chill until serving.

Nutrition: 255 Calories: 15g Protein: 19g Carbohydrates

Crispy Zucchini Fritters

Preparation: 15 min | Cooking: 20 min | Servings: 6

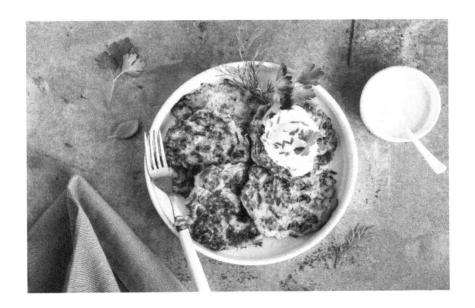

Ingredients

- 2 large green zucchinis
- 1 cup flour
- 1 large egg, beaten
- ½ cup water
- 1 teaspoon baking powder

Directions

1. Grate the zucchini into a large bowl.

2. Add the 2 tbsp. of parsley, 3 garlic cloves, salt, flour, egg, water, and baking powder to the bowl and stir to combine.
3. In a large pot or fryer over medium heat, heat oil to 365°F.
4. Drop the fritter batter into 3 cups of vegetable oil. Turn the fritters over using a slotted spoon and fry until they are golden brown, about 2 to 3 min.
5. Strain fritters from the oil and place on a plate lined with paper towels.
6. Serve warm with Creamy Tzatziki or Creamy Traditional Hummus as a dip.

Nutrition: 446 Calories: 5g Protein: 19g Carbohydrates

Green Beans and Potatoes in Olive Oil

Preparation: 12 min | Cooking: 17 min | Servings: 4

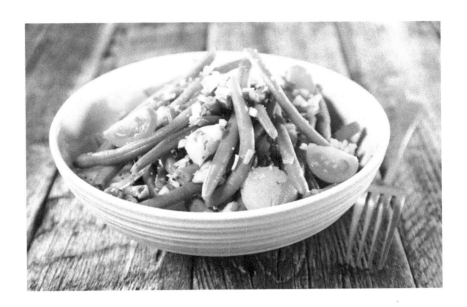

Ingredients

- 15 oz. tomatoes (diced)
- 2 potatoes
- 1 lb. green beans (fresh)
- 1 bunch dill, parsley, zucchini
- 1 tbsp. dried oregano

Directions

1. Turn on the sauté function on your instant pot.

2. Pour tomatoes, a cup of water and olive oil. Stir in the rest of the ingredients and stir through.
3. Close the instant pot and click the valve to seal. Set time for fifteen min.
4. When the time has elapsed release pressure. Remove the Fasolakia from the instant pot. Serve and enjoy.

Nutrition: 510 Calories: 20g Protein: 28g Carbohydrates

Cheesy Spinach Pies

Preparation: 20 min | Cooking: 40 min | Servings: 5

Ingredients

- 2 tablespoons extra-virgin olive oil
- 3 (1-pound) bags of baby spinach, washed
- 1 cup feta cheese
- 1 large egg, beaten
- Puff pastry sheets

Directions

1. Preheat the oven to 375°F.
2. Using big skillet over medium heat, cook the olive oil, 1 onion, and 2 garlic cloves for 3 min.
3. Add the spinach to the skillet one bag at a time, letting it wilt in between each bag. Toss using tongs. Cook for 4 min. Once cooked, strain any extra liquid from the pan.
4. Mix feta cheese, egg, and cooked spinach.
5. Lay the puff pastry flat on a counter. Cut the pastry into 3-inch squares.
6. Place a tablespoon of the spinach mixture in the center of a puff-pastry square. Turn over one corner of the square to the diagonal corner,

forming a triangle. Crimp the edges of the pie by pressing down with the tines of a fork to seal them together. Repeat until all squares are filled.

7. Situate the pies on a parchment-lined baking sheet and bake for 25 to 30 min or until golden brown. Serve warm or at room temperature.

Nutrition: 503 Calories: 16g Protein: 38g Carbohydrates

Pot Black Eyed Peas

Preparation: 6 min | Cooking: 25 min | Servings: 4

Ingredients

- 2 cups black-eyed peas (dried)
- 1 cup parsley, dill
- 2 slices oranges
- 2 tbsp. tomato paste
- 4 green onions
- 2 carrots, bay leaves

Directions

1. Clean the dill thoroughly with water removing stones.
2. Add all the ingredients in the instant pot and stir well to combine.
3. Lid the instant pot and set the vent to sealing.
4. Set time for twenty-five min. When the time has elapsed release pressure naturally.
5. Serve and enjoy the black-eyed peas.

Nutrition: 506 Calories: 14g Protein: 33g Carbohydrates

Nutritious Vegan Cabbage

Preparation: 35 min | Cooking: 15 min | Servings: 6

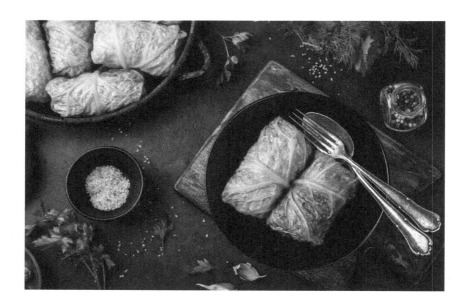

Ingredients

- 3 cups green cabbage
- 1 can tomatoes, onion
- Cups vegetable broth
- 3 stalks celery, carrots
- 2 tbsp. vinegar, sage

Directions

1. Mix 1 tbsp. of lemon juice. 2 garlic cloves and the rest of ingredients in the instant pot and. Lid and set time for fifteen min on high pressure.
2. Release pressure naturally then remove the lid. Remove the soup from the instant pot.
3. Serve and enjoy.

Nutrition: 67 Calories: 0.4g Fat 3.8g Fiber

Instant Pot Horta and Potatoes

Preparation: 12 min | Cooking: 17 min | Servings: 4

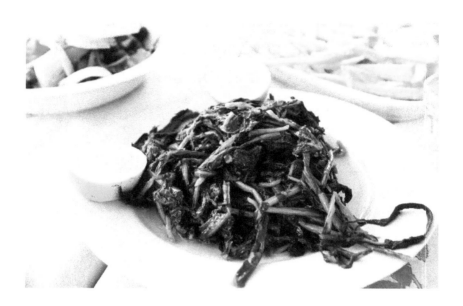

Ingredients

- 2 heads of washed and chopped greens (spinach, Dandelion, kale, mustard green, Swiss chard)
- 6 potatoes (washed and cut in pieces)
- 1 cup virgin olive oil
- 1 lemon juice (reserve slices for serving)
- 10 garlic cloves (chopped)

Directions

1. Position all the ingredients in the instant pot and lid setting the vent to sealing.
2. Set time for fifteen min. When time is done release pressure.
3. Let the potatoes rest for some time. Serve and enjoy with lemon slices.

Nutrition: 499 Calories: 18g Protein: 41g Carbohydrates

Instant Pot Artichokes with Mediterranean Aioli

Preparation: 7 min | Cooking: 10 min | Servings: 3

Ingredients

- 3 medium artichokes (stems cut off)
- 1 cup vegetable broth
- Mediterranean aioli

Directions

1. Place wire trivet in place in the instant pot then place the artichokes on the wire.
2. Pour vegetable broth over artichokes.
3. Lid the instant pot and put steam mode on. Set time for 10 min. When the time has elapsed allow pressure to release.
4. Remove the artichokes from the instant pot and reserve the remaining broth, about a quarter cup.
5. Half the artichokes and place them on serving bowls. Drizzle broth.
6. Serve with aioli and enjoy.

Nutrition: 30 Calories: 0.1g Fat 3.5g Fiber

Instant Pot Jackfruit Curry

Preparation: 1 h | Cooking: 16 min | Servings: 2

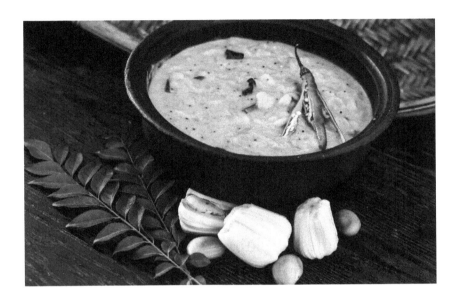

Ingredients

- 1 tbsp. oil
- Cumin seeds, Mustard seeds
- 2 tomatoes (purred)
- 20 oz. can green jackfruit (drained and rinsed)
- 1 tbsp. coriander powder, turmeric.

Directions

1. Turn the instant pot to sauté mode. Add cumin seeds, mustard, ten nigella seeds and allow them to sizzle.
2. Add 2 red chilies and 2 bay leaves and allow cooking for a few seconds.
3. Add chopped 1 onion, 5 garlic cloves, ginger and salt, and pepper to taste. Stir cook for five min.
4. Add other ingredients and a cup of water then lid the instant pot. Set time for seven min on high pressure.
5. When the time has elapsed release pressure naturally, shred the jackfruit and serve.

Nutrition: 369 Calories: 3g Fat 6g Fiber

Red Wine Risotto

Servings: 8 | Cooking: 25 min

Ingredients

- Pepper to taste
- 1 cup finely shredded Parmigian-Reggiano cheese, divided
- 2 tsp tomato paste
- 1 ¾ cups dry red wine
- ¼ tsp salt
- 1 ½ cups Italian 'risotto' rice
- 2 cloves garlic, minced
- 1 medium onion, freshly chopped
- 2 tbsp extra-virgin olive oil
- 4 ½ cups reduced sodium beef broth

Directions

1. On medium high fire, bring to a simmer broth in a medium fry pan. Lower fire so broth is steaming but not simmering.
2. On medium low heat, place a Dutch oven and heat oil.

3. Sauté onions for 5 minutes. Add garlic and cook for 2 minutes.
4. Add rice, mix well, and season with salt.
5. Into rice, add a generous splash of wine and ½ cup of broth.
6. Lower fire to a gentle simmer, cook until liquid is fully absorbed while stirring rice every once in a while.
7. Add another splash of wine and ½ cup of broth. Stirring once in a while.
8. Add tomato paste and stir to mix well.
9. Continue cooking and adding wine and broth until broth is used up.
10. Once done cooking, turn off fire and stir in pepper and ¾ cup cheese.
11. To serve, sprinkle with remaining cheese and enjoy.

Nutrition: Calories: 231; Carbs: 33.9g; Protein: 7.9g; Fat: 5.7g

Chicken Pasta Parmesan

Servings: 1 | Cooking: 20 min

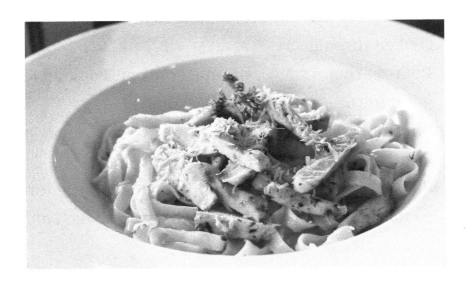

Ingredients

- ¼ cup prepared marinara sauce
- ½ cup cooked whole wheat spaghetti
- 1 oz reduced fat mozzarella cheese, grated
- 1 tbsp olive oil
- 2 tbsp seasoned dry breadcrumbs
- 4 oz skinless chicken breast

Directions

1. On medium high fire, place an ovenproof skillet and heat oil.
2. Pan fry chicken for 3 to 5 minutes per side or until cooked through.
3. Pour marinara sauce, stir and continue cooking for 3 minutes.
4. Turn off fire, add mozzarella and breadcrumbs on top.
5. Pop into a preheated broiler on high and broil for 10 minutes or until breadcrumbs are browned and mozzarella is melted.
6. Remove from broiler, serve and enjoy.

Nutrition: Calories: 529; Carbs: 34.4g; Protein: 38g; Fat: 26.6g

Tasty Lasagna Rolls

Servings: 6 | Cooking: 20 min

Ingredients

- ¼ tsp crushed red pepper
- ¼ tsp salt
- ½ cup shredded mozzarella cheese
- ½ cups parmesan cheese, shredded
- 1 14-oz package tofu, cubed
- 1 25-oz can of low-sodium marinara sauce
- 1 tbsp extra virgin olive oil
- 12 whole wheat lasagna noodles
- 2 tbsp Kalamata olives, chopped
- 3 cloves minced garlic
- 3 cups spinach, chopped

Directions

1. Put enough water on a large pot and cook the lasagna noodles according to package instructions. Drain, rinse and set aside until ready to use.

2. In a large skillet, sauté garlic over medium heat for 20 seconds. Add the tofu and spinach and cook until the spinach wilts. Transfer this mixture in a

bowl and add parmesan olives, salt, red pepper and 2/3 cup of the marinara sauce.

3. In a pan, spread a cup of marinara sauce on the bottom. To make the rolls, place noodle on a surface and spread ¼ cup of the tofu filling. Roll up and place it on the pan with the marinara sauce. Do this procedure until all lasagna noodles are rolled.

4. Place the pan over high heat and bring to a simmer. Reduce the heat to medium and let it cook for three more minutes. Sprinkle mozzarella cheese and let the cheese melt for two minutes. Serve hot.

Nutrition: Calories: 304; Carbs: 39.2g; Protein: 23g; Fat: 19.2g

Raisins, Nuts And Beef On Hashweh Rice

Servings: 8 | Cooking: 50 min

Ingredients

- ½ cup dark raisins, soaked in 2 cups water for an hour
- 1/3 cup slivered almonds, toasted and soaked in 2 cups water overnight
- 1/3 cup pine nuts, toasted and soaked in 2 cups water overnight
- ½ cup fresh parsley leaves, roughly chopped
- Pepper and salt to taste
- ¾ tsp ground cinnamon, divided
- ¾ tsp cloves, divided
- 1 tsp garlic powder
- 1 ¾ tsp allspice, divided
- 1 lb. lean ground beef or lean ground lamb
- 1 small red onion, finely chopped
- Olive oil
- 1 ½ cups medium grain rice

Directions

1. For 15 to 20 minutes, soak rice in cold water. You will know that soaking is enough when you can snap a grain of rice easily between your thumb and index finger. Once soaking is done, drain rice well.

2. Meanwhile, drain pine nuts, almonds and raisins for at least a minute and transfer to one bowl. Set aside.

3. On a heavy cooking pot on medium high fire, heat 1 tbsp olive oil.

4. Once oil is hot, add red onions. Sauté for a minute before adding ground meat and sauté for another minute.

5. Season ground meat with pepper, salt, ½ tsp ground cinnamon, ½ tsp ground cloves, 1 tsp garlic powder, and 1 ¼ tsp allspice.

6. Sauté ground meat for 10 minutes or until browned and cooked fully. Drain fat.

7. In same pot with cooked ground meat, add rice on top of meat.

8. Season with a bit of pepper and salt. Add remaining cinnamon, ground cloves, and allspice. Do not mix.

9. Add 1 tbsp olive oil and 2 ½ cups of water. Bring to a boil and once boiling, lower fire to a simmer. Cook while covered until liquid is fully absorbed, around 20 to 25 minutes.

10. Turn of fire.

11. To serve, place a large serving platter that fully covers the mouth of the pot. Place platter upside down on mouth of pot, and invert pot. The inside of the pot should now rest on the platter with the rice on bottom of plate and ground meat on top of it.

12. Garnish the top of the meat with raisins, almonds, pine nuts, and parsley.

13. Serve and enjoy.

Nutrition: Calories per serving: 357; Carbs: 39.0g; Protein: 16.7g; Fat: 15.9g

Yangchow Chinese Style Fried Rice

Servings: 4 | Cooking: 20 min

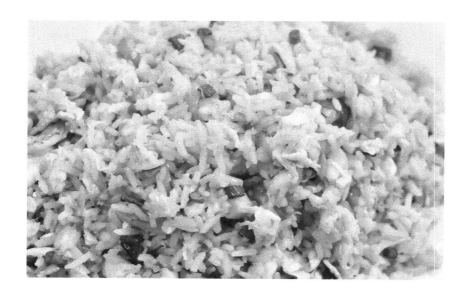

Ingredients

- 4 cups cold cooked rice
- 1/2 cup peas
- 1 medium yellow onion, diced
- 5 tbsp olive oil
- 4 oz frozen medium shrimp, thawed, shelled, deveined and chopped finely
- 6 oz roast pork
- 3 large eggs

- Salt and freshly ground black pepper
- 1/2 tsp cornstarch

Directions

1. Combine the salt and ground black pepper and 1/2 tsp cornstarch, coat the shrimp with it. Chop the roasted pork. Beat the eggs and set aside.

2. Stir-fry the shrimp in a wok on high fire with 1 tbsp heated oil until pink, around 3 minutes. Set the shrimp aside and stir fry the roasted pork briefly. Remove both from the pan.

3. In the same pan, stir-fry the onion until soft, Stir the peas and cook until bright green. Remove both from pan.

4. Add 2 tbsp oil in the same pan, add the cooked rice. Stir and separate the individual grains. Add the beaten eggs, toss the rice. Add the roasted pork, shrimp, vegetables and onion. Toss everything together. Season with salt and pepper to taste.

Nutrition: Calories per serving: 556; Carbs: 60.2g; Protein: 20.2g; Fat: 25.2g

Chapter 7: Dessert Recipes

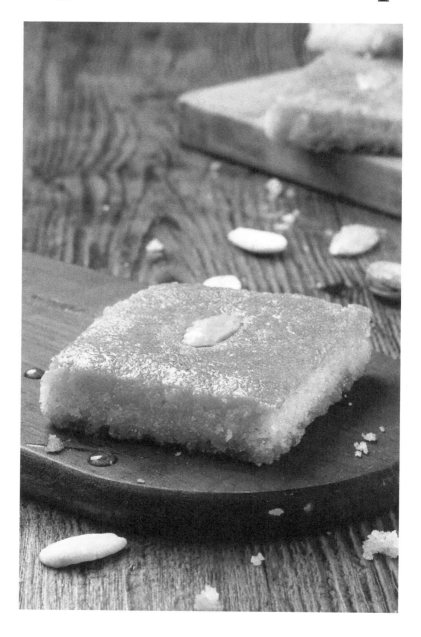

White Wine Grapefruit Poached Peaches

Servings: 6 | Cooking: 40 min

Ingredients

- 4 peaches
- 2 cups white wine
- 1 grapefruit, peeled and juiced
- ¼ cup white sugar
- 1 cinnamon stick
- 1 star anise
- 1 cardamom pod
- 1 cup Greek yogurt for serving

Directions

1. Combine the wine, grapefruit, sugar and spices in a saucepan.
2. Bring to a boil then place the peaches in the hot syrup.
3. Lower the heat and cover with a lid. Cook for 15 minutes then allow to cool down.
4. Carefully peel the peaches and place them in a small serving bowl.

5. Top with yogurt and serve right away.

Nutrition: Calories:157 Fat:0.9g Protein:4.2g
Carbohydrates:20.4g

Cinnamon Stuffed Peaches

Servings: 4 | Cooking: 5 min

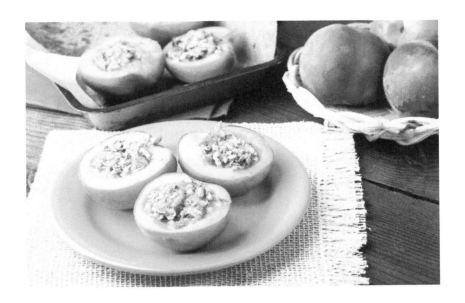

Ingredients

- 4 peaches, pitted, halved
- 2 tablespoons ricotta cheese
- 2 tablespoons of liquid honey
- ¾ cup of water
- ½ teaspoon vanilla extract
- ¾ teaspoon ground cinnamon
- 1 tablespoon almonds, sliced
- ¾ teaspoon saffron

Directions

1. Pour water in the saucepan and bring to boil.
2. Add vanilla extract, saffron, ground cinnamon, and liquid honey.
3. Cook the liquid until the honey is melted.
4. Then remove it from the heat.
5. Put the halved peaches in the hot honey liquid.
6. Meanwhile, make the filling: mix up together ricotta cheese, vanilla extract, and sliced almonds.
7. Remove the peaches from honey liquid and arrange in the plate.
8. Fill 4 peach halves with ricotta filling and cover them with remaining peach halves.
9. Sprinkle the cooked dessert with liquid honey mixture gently.

Nutrition: calories 113; fat 1.8; fiber 2.8; carbs 23.9; protein 2.7

Eggless Farina Cake (namoura)

Servings: 1 Piece | Cooking: 40 min

Ingredients

- 2 cups farina
- 1/2 cup semolina
- 1/2 cup all-purpose flour
- 1 TB. baking powder
- 1 tsp. active dry yeast
- 1/2 cup sugar
- 1/2 cup plain Greek yogurt
- 1 cup whole milk
- 3/4 cup butter, melted
- 1/4 cup water
- 2 TB. tahini paste
- 15 almonds
- 2 cups Simple Syrup

Directions

1. In a large bowl, combine farina, semolina, all-purpose flour, baking powder, yeast, sugar, Greek yogurt, whole milk, butter, and water. Set aside for 15 minutes.

2. Preheat the oven to 375°F.

3. Spread tahini paste evenly in the bottom of a 9×13-inch baking pan, and pour in cake batter. Arrange almonds on top of batter, about where each slice will be. Bake for 45 minutes or until golden brown.

4. Remove cake from the oven, and using a toothpick, poke holes throughout cake for Simple Syrup to seep into. Pour syrup over cake, and let cake sit for 1 hour to absorb syrup.

5. Cool cake completely before cutting and serving.

Banana And Berries Trifle

Servings: 10 | Cooking: 5 min

Ingredients

- 8 oz biscuits, chopped
- ¼ cup strawberries, chopped
- 1 banana, chopped
- 1 peach, chopped
- ½ mango, chopped
- 1 cup grapes, chopped
- 1 tablespoon liquid honey
- 1 cup of orange juice
- ½ cup Plain yogurt
- ¼ cup cream cheese
- 1 teaspoon coconut flakes

Directions

1. Bring the orange juice to boil and remove it from the heat.
2. Add liquid honey and stir until it is dissolved.
3. Cool the liquid to the room temperature.

4. Add chopped banana, peach, mango, grapes, and strawberries. Shake the fruits gently and leave to soak the orange juice for 15 minutes.
5. Meanwhile, with the help of the hand mixer mix up together Plain yogurt and cream cheese.
6. Then separate the chopped biscuits, yogurt mixture, and fruits on 4 parts.
7. Place the first part of biscuits in the big serving glass in one layer.
8. Spread it with yogurt mixture and add fruits.
9. Repeat the same steps till you use all ingredients.
10.   Top the trifle with coconut flakes.

Nutrition: calories 164; fat 6.2; fiber 1.3; carbs 24.8; protein 3.2

Mixed Berry Sorbet

Servings: 8 | Cooking: 2 ½ Hours

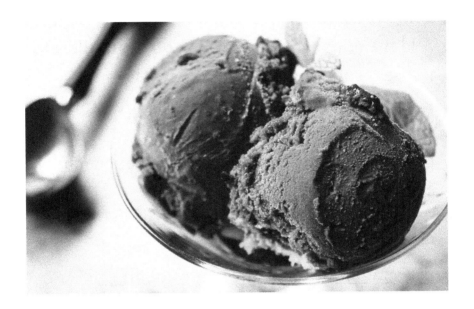

Ingredients

- 2 cups water
- ½ cup white sugar
- 2 cups mixed berries
- 1 tablespoon lemon juice
- 2 tablespoons honey
- 1 teaspoon lemon zest
- 1 mint sprig

Directions

1. Combine the water, sugar, berries, lemon juice, honey and lemon zest in a saucepan.
2. Bring to a boil and cook on low heat for 5 minutes.
3. Add the mint sprig and remove off heat. Allow to infuse for 10 minutes then remove the mint.
4. Pour the syrup into a blender and puree until smooth and creamy.
5. Pour the smooth syrup into an airtight container and freeze for at least 2 hours.
6. Serve the sorbet chilled.

Nutrition: Calories:84 Fat:0.1g Protein:0.4g Carbohydrates:21.3g

CPSIA information can be obtained
at www.ICGtesting.com
Printed in the USA
BVHW090851140621
609525BV00002B/60

9 781803 257037